Safety First

HOME

By Cynthia Fitterer Klingel
Pictures by Tom Dunnington

Creative Education, Inc.
Mankato, Minnesota 56001

Published by Creative Education, Inc.,
123 South Broad Street, Mankato, Minnesota 56001
Copyright © 1986 by Creative Education, Inc.
International copyrights reserved in all countries.
No part of this book may be reproduced in any form without
written permission from the publisher.
Printed in the United States.

Library of Congress Cataloging in Publication Data
Klingel, Cynthia Fitterer
    SAFETY FIRST ... HOME.
    SUMMARY: Simple text and illustrations point
out rules to follow in order to avoid accidents
in the home.
    1. Home accidents—Prevention—Juvenile
literature. [1. Accidents] I. Dunnington, Tom.
II. Title.
TX150.B34   614.8'53   79-25796   ISBN 0-87191-739-4

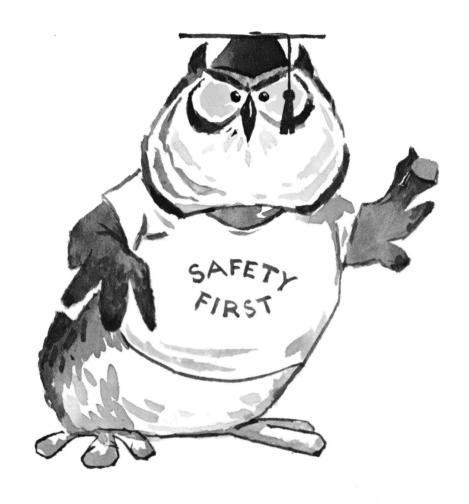

"Hi! I'm Ollie the Safety Owl. I have been busy helping my friends, Rover, the cat, and Basil, the dog, play safely. Today they are home from school. What do you think they will find to do? I hope they remember our safety rules!" I'd better check on them to make sure!

"I am the world's best cook," remarked Basil. "What would you like me to make for you?"

Rover just smiled. He had tasted Basil's cooking before!

Suddenly, something smelled like it was burning. Basil and Rover didn't even notice.

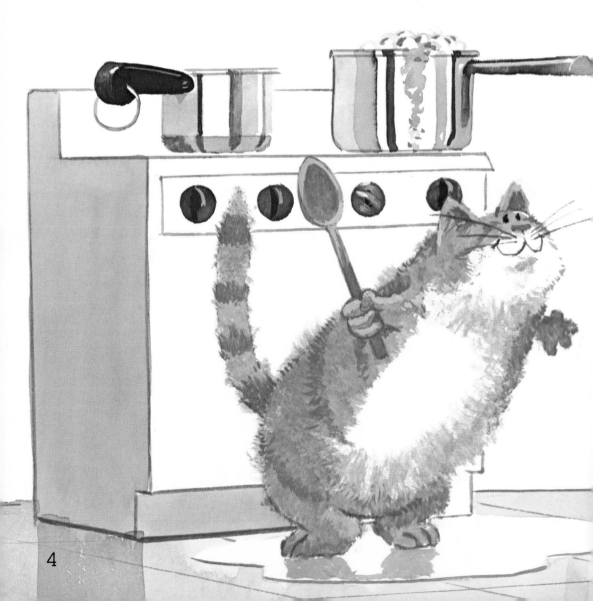

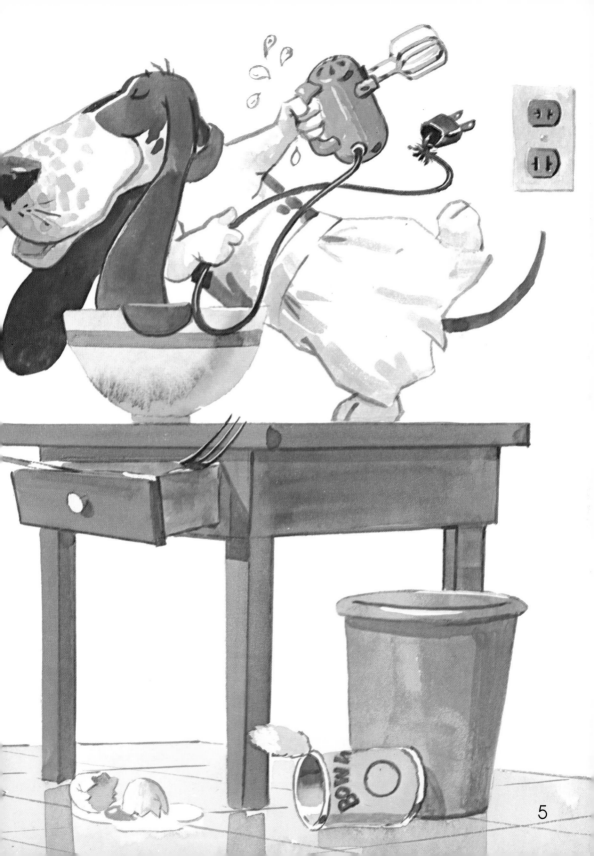

5

But Ollie smelled it and rushed over.

"What a mess!" Ollie cried. "We need to clean it up right away."

When working in the kitchen, remember these rules:

- Make sure electric machines are in good shape.
- Do not touch electric machines with wet hands.
- Use the plug, not the cord to unplug electrical machines.

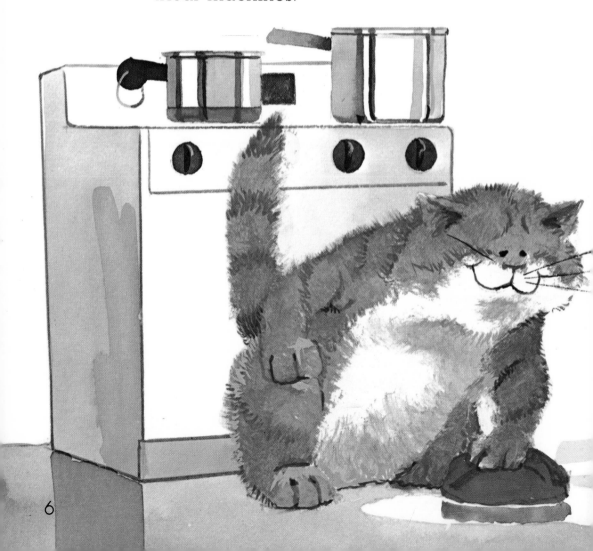

- Wipe up liquids spilled on the floor.
- Have help with sharp kitchen tools.
- Be careful of sharp can covers.
- Turn pot handles to the back of the stove.
- Watch anything that is cooking on the stove.

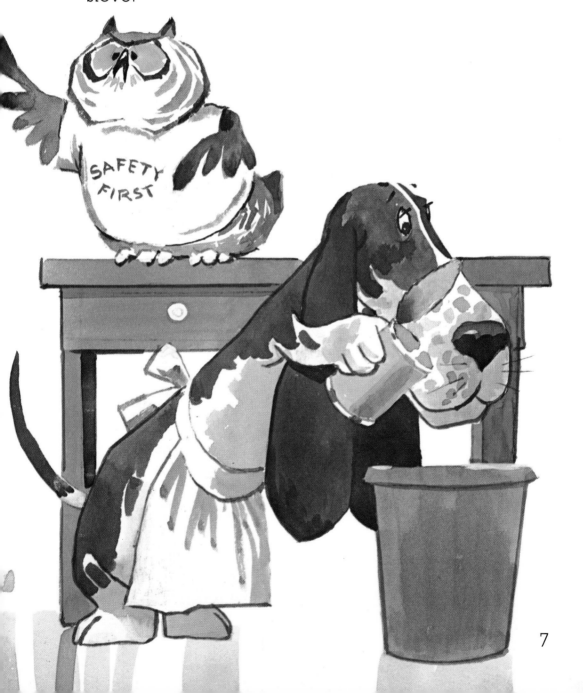

"Come on, Rover. Let's play tag. You're It," said Basil.

"No, Basil. This isn't a safe way to play. I think we should pick things up," answered Rover.

So they did.

They closed the gate at the top of the stairs. They picked up the toys on the stairs. Rover put away the raincoat and umbrella.

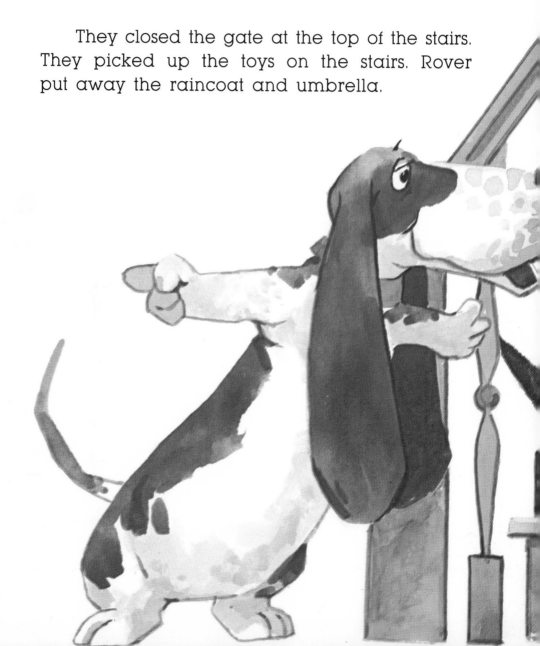

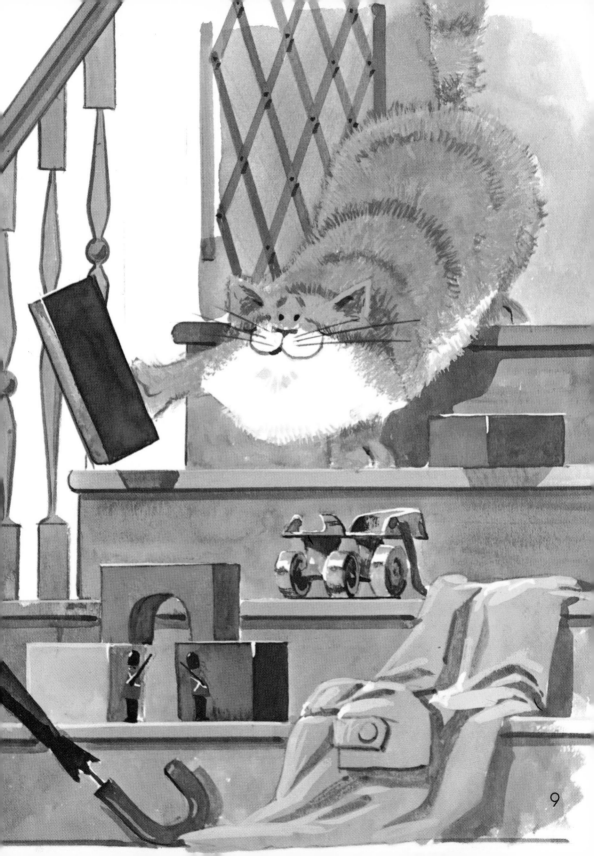

Just then Ollie flew in the door.
"I'm so proud of you," said Ollie.
Rover and Basil smiled.

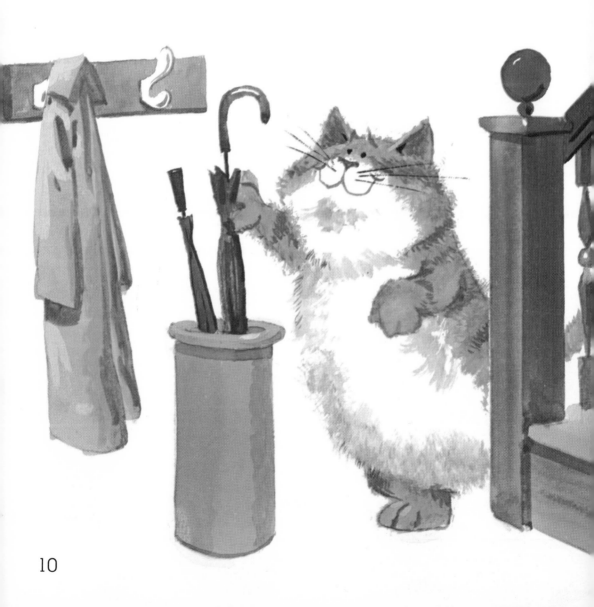

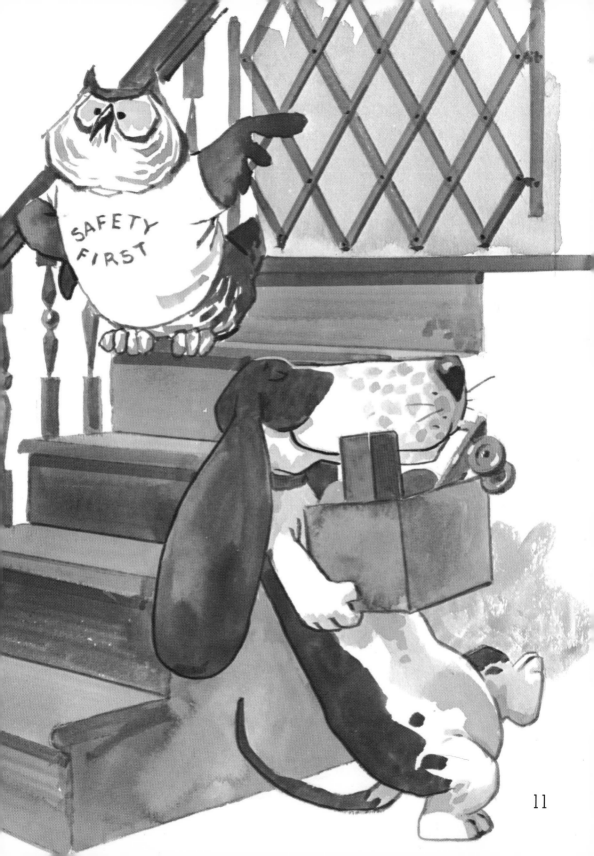

11

But a few minutes later, they forgot all about playing safely.

"Jump, jump," cried Basil. "You'll never catch me."

"Yes, I will," answered Rover. "Whee-e-e-e, here I come."

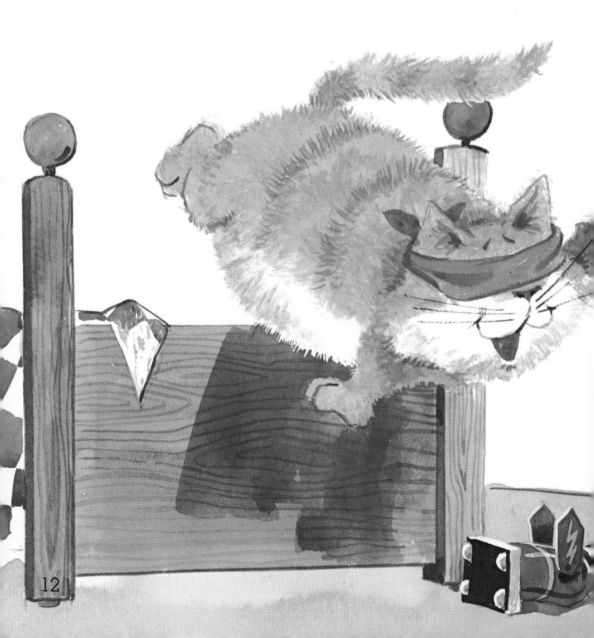

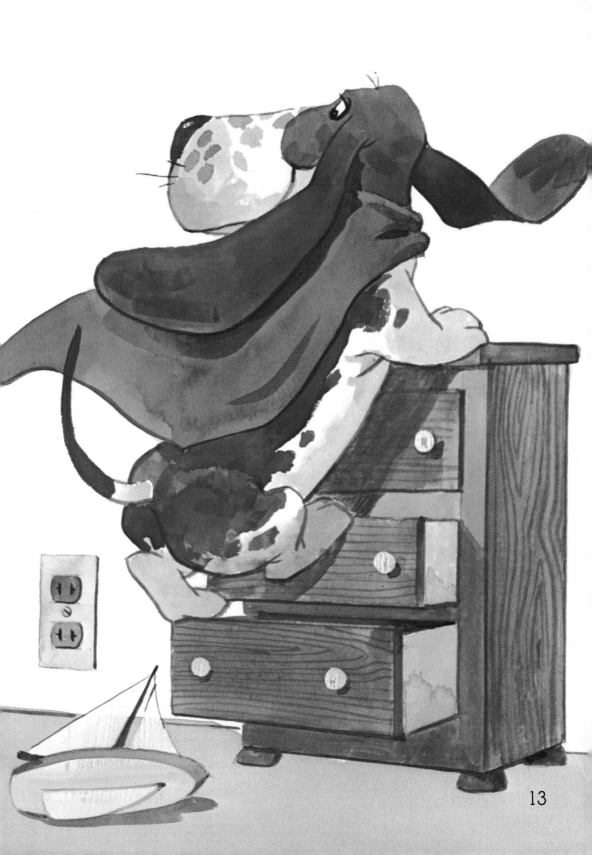

13

In flew Ollie.

"Oh, my!" cried Ollie. "What are you up to now?"

"We were having fun!" shouted Rover.

"Fun!" said Ollie. "Rover, never play with your eyes closed or covered, and Basil, you should never climb on furniture. What else did you forget?"

"We forgot to watch for sharp objects and to put toys away so we don't trip on them," answered Basil.

"Right!" said Ollie.

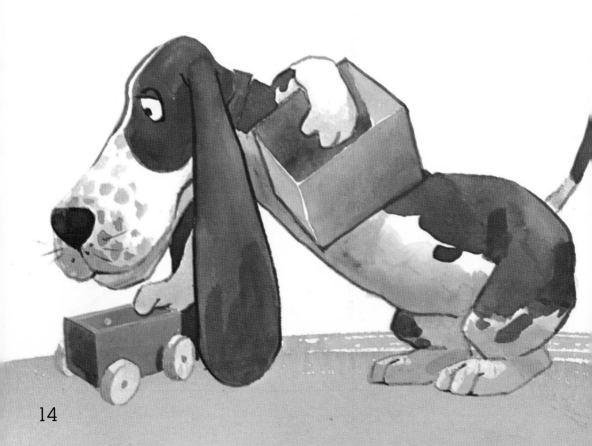

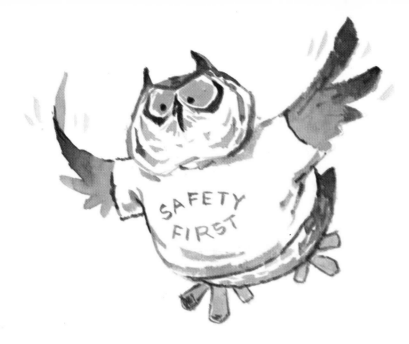

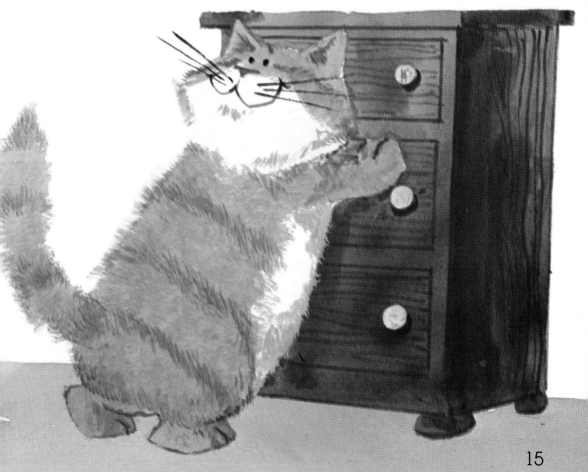

"Let's not make a mess anymore," said Rover. "Hey, look! I can fit in this plastic bag!"

"I'll play with that gun while you play in the plastic bag," answered Basil.

Are Rover and Basil being good thinkers?

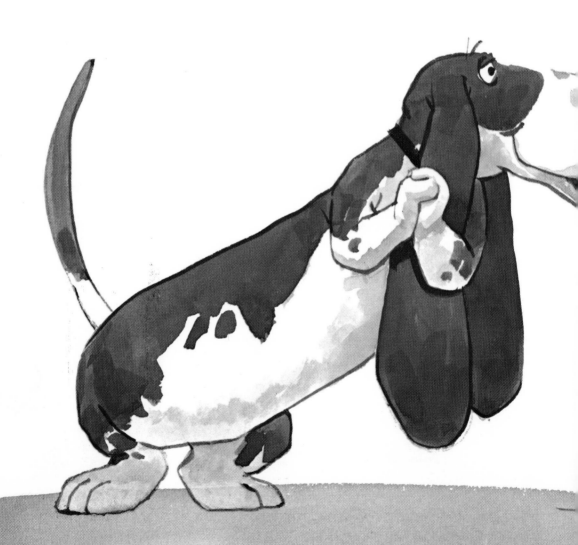

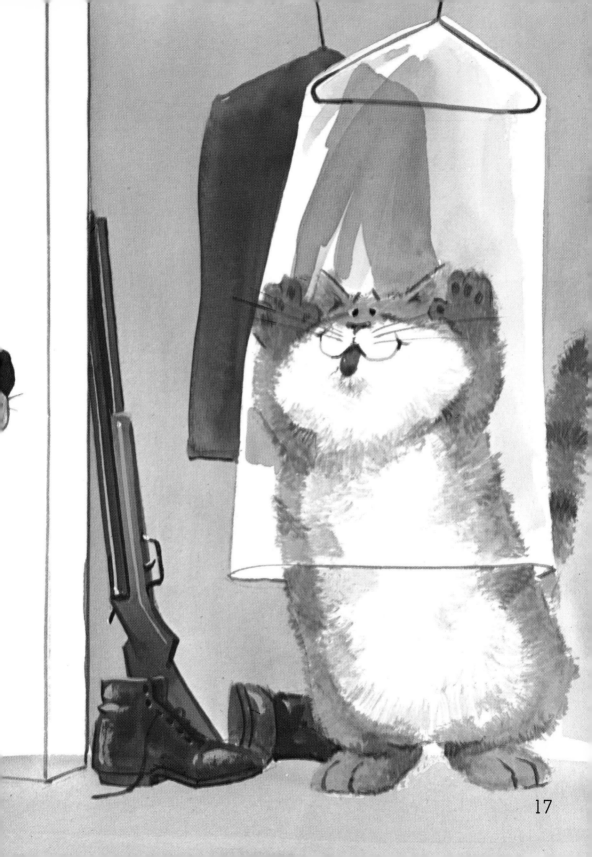

17

No! They are not!

"Stop!" cried Ollie. "NEVER touch or play with guns. And never play with plastic bags. They can be very dangerous! You two are lucky I came before anything happened!"

"Thank you for helping us, Ollie," said Rover.

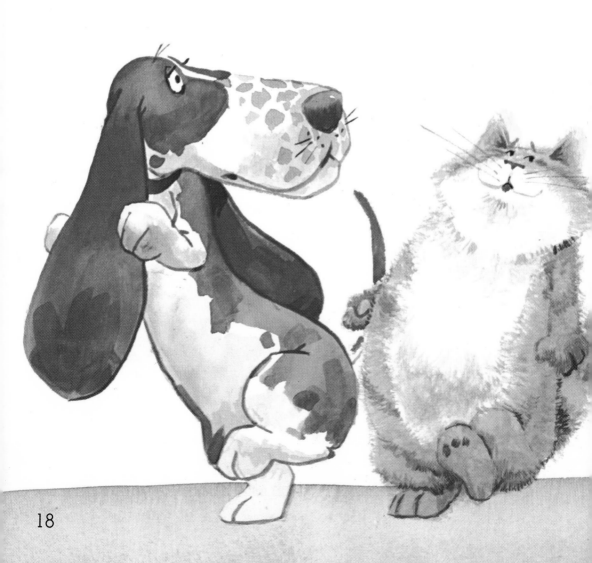

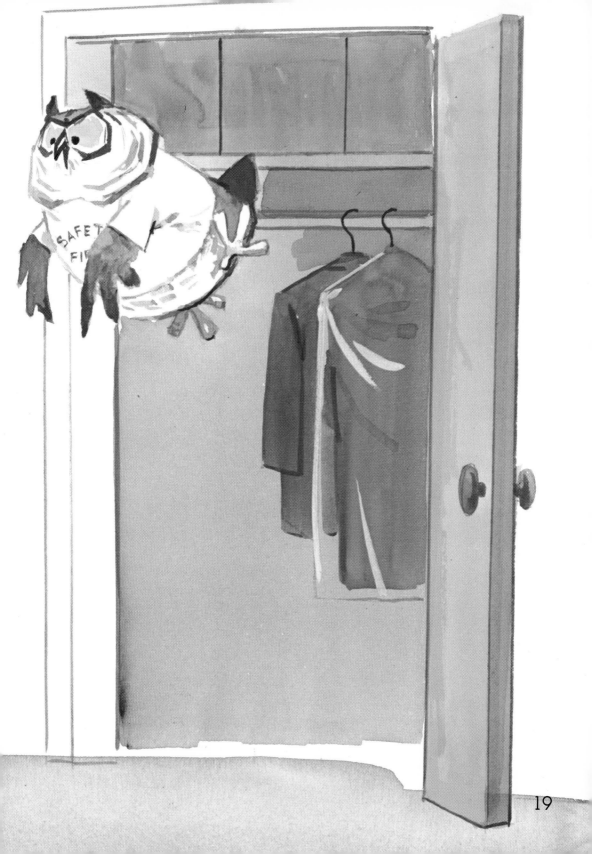

19

"I'm going in for a swim," laughed Rover.

"Here, use the blow dryer to fluff your fur. Do you want to brush your teeth while you're in the water?" asked Basil.

Do you think that's a good idea?

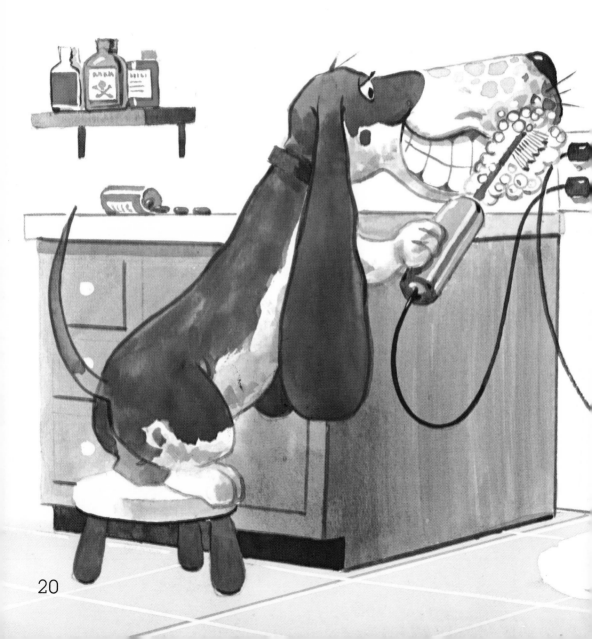

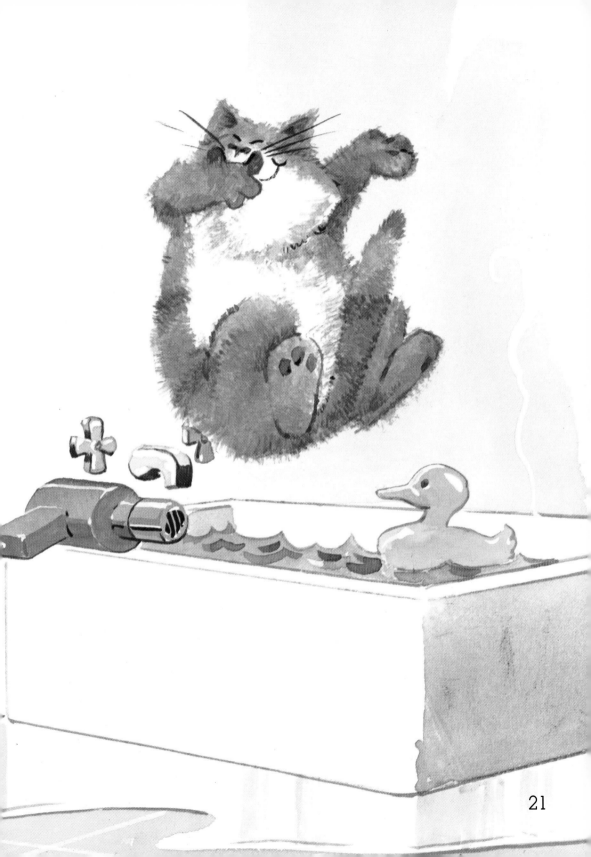

"That's not a good idea," said Ollie.
Remember these safety rules:
- Use a rubber mat in the tub or shower.
- Check water in tub to see if it is too hot.
- Keep electrical machines away from water.
- Keep floor dry.
- Medicine should be kept in a cupboard away from small children.

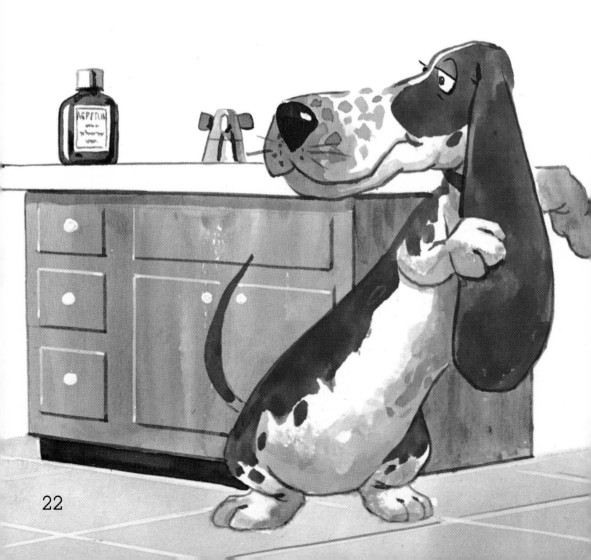

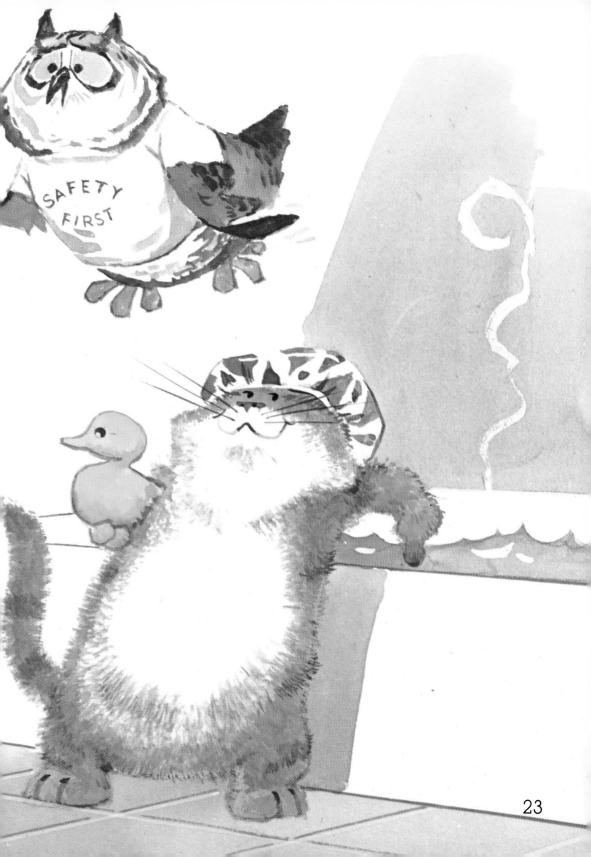

23

"Hi, Basil. I didn't think you'd find me in here," said Rover.

"Your tail was sticking out," answered Basil. "This place is really a mess. It's not very safe."

"Really? What's wrong?" asked Rover.

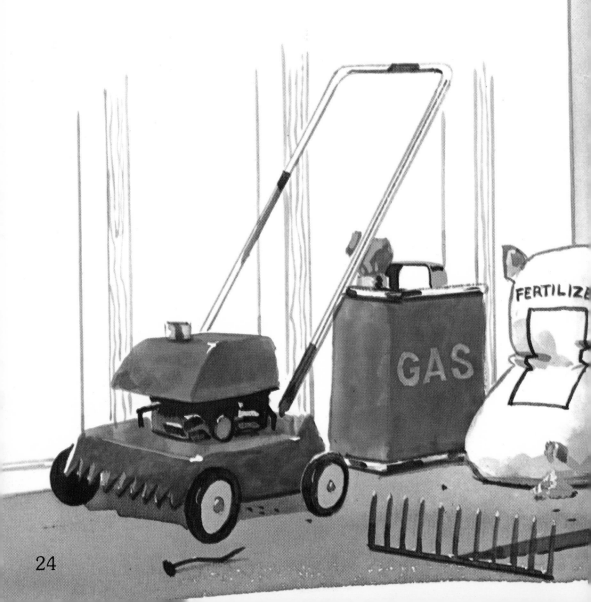

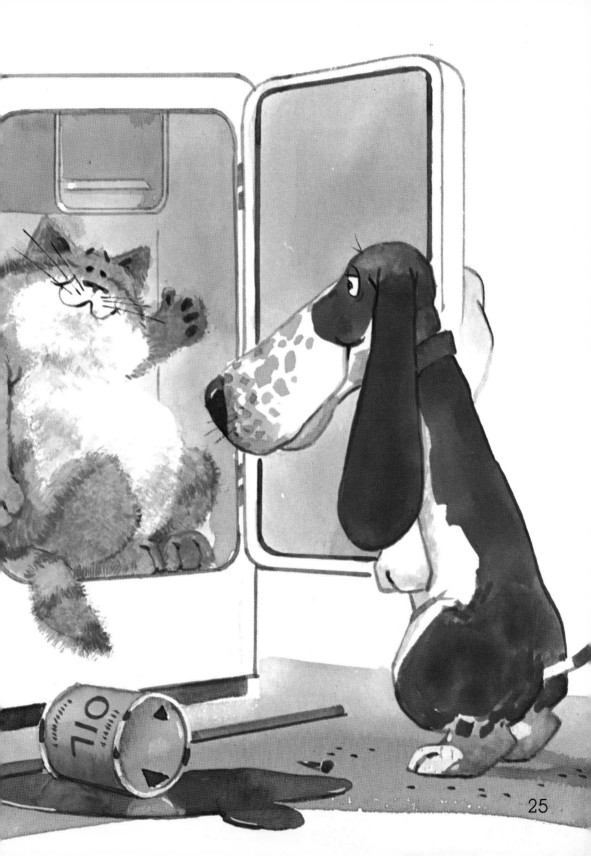

25

"Don't play with garden tools — they are very sharp. Don't touch or play with poison — like gas, oil, or fertilizer. Keep the floor clean," answered Basil.

"And never play inside an empty trunk or refrigerator," added Ollie.

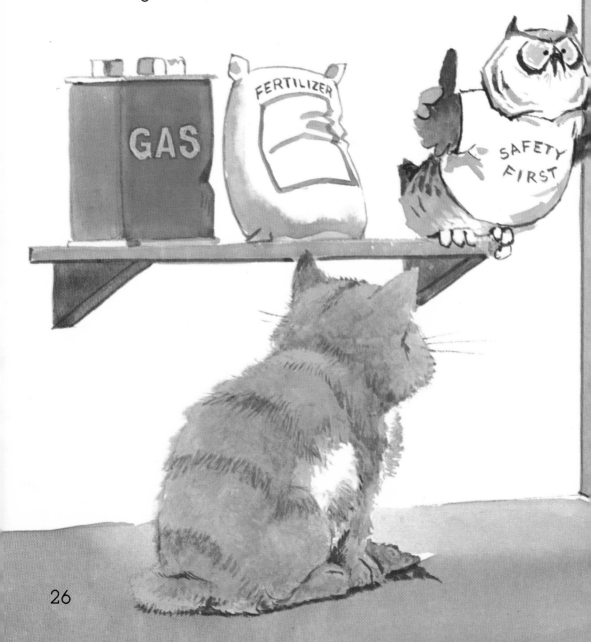

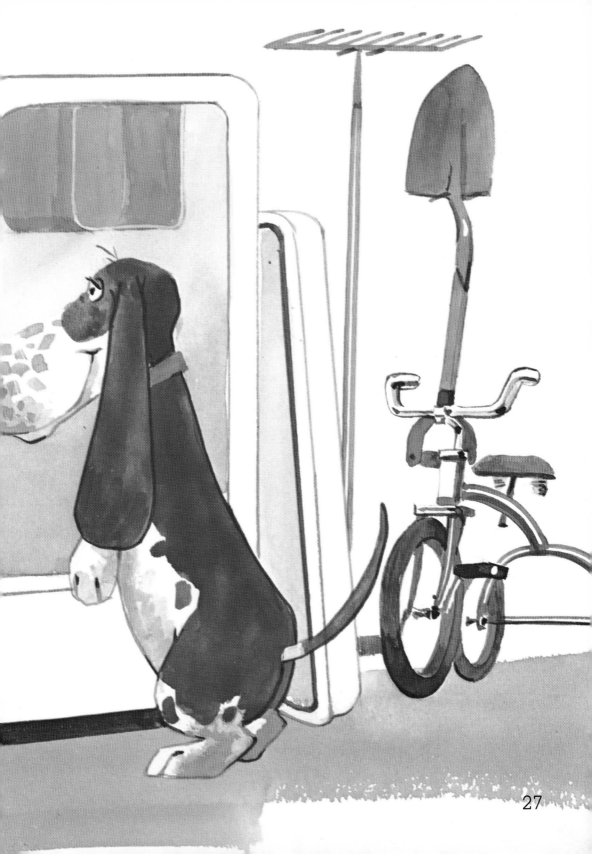

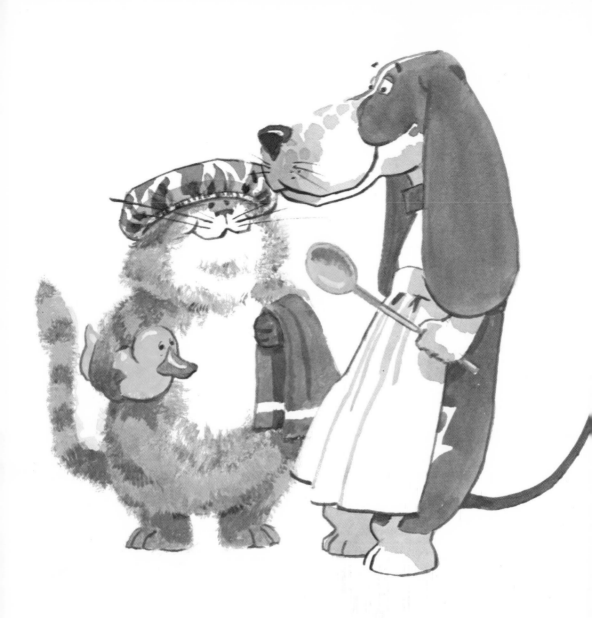

Rover and Basil thought about their day. They had learned a lot about how to play safely at home. Let's see if you can remember the safety rules they learned today:

28

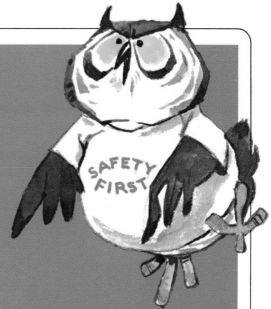

- Make sure electric machines are in good shape.
- Do not touch electric machines with wet hands.
- Use the plug, not the cord, to unplug electric machines.
- Wipe up liquid spilled on the floor.
- Have help with sharp kitchen tools.
- Be careful of sharp can covers.
- Turn pot handles to back of stove.
- Watch anything that is cooking on the stove.

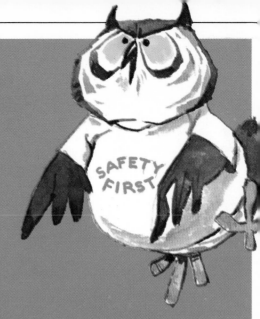

- Keep stairway gates locked.
- Do not leave toys on stairway.
- Hang up coat and umbrella.

- Don't play with your eyes closed.
- Don't climb on furniture.
- Watch out for sharp cabinet corners.
- Put toys away so you don't trip over them.

- Do NOT touch guns!
- Don't play with plastic cleaning bags.

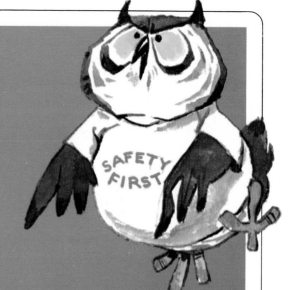

- Use a rubber mat in the tub or shower.
- Check water in tub to see if it is too hot.
- Keep floor dry.
- Keep electrical hair dryers away from water.
- Medicine should be kept in a cupboard away from small children.

- Don't play with garden tools.
- Don't touch or play with poison — like gas, oil or fertilizer.
- Keep floor clean.
- Never get inside an empty trunk or refrigerator.